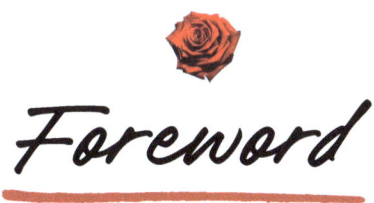

Foreword

This workbook has been a long time coming. I have always wanted to create a body of work to help people through their toughest moments. This work is the sum of all the things I have learned going through breakups, and more recently the end of my marriage. As my grandmother remarked, "you are such a pretty girl, but you don't know how to pick them."

I offer this to my fellow women and men who may have a broken picker. May this book take you on a journey of healing, self-reflection, incredible insight, and most of all hope, hope that one day you will meet and have endless love with your person.

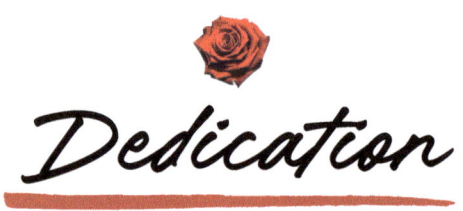

Dedication

I first dedicate this book to God, the one who never left my side, may I continue to sit at your feet. To my mother and father, thank you for raising me to feel unstoppable. To my brother thank you for always protecting me and supporting me. To my besties......thank you. To my son, may you take this work as an example that nothing in life is too hard to achieve when you have God at the head of your life.

Scan the code to watch an introductory video on how to use this workbook, or visit www.lavantedorsey.com.

Table of Contents

Is It Really

OVER?

Is it Really Over?

As I sat processing the current state of marriage. As I sat in the disconnect, the poor communication, the constant arguing, and the lack of romance and love. I wondered; how did we get here? The last 8 years we had meant so much to each other. Yet current day, connection was a hit or miss. I was tired, I had no more fight left in me, it was time to face the reality. It was really over. A lot of times the hardest part is accepting that the relationship we thought we had is not the one we are living in, as well as accepting that the relationship is beyond repair. Perhaps too much damage has occurred, or the hard truth that you and your partner have grown apart. The values you once shared may no longer complement each other. Perhaps there has been infidelity, abuse, or just plain old toxicity.

Whatever the reason, I would assume you purchased this book because there is a piece of you that recognized that you deserve so much more. There is a piece of you which knows that staying in a relationship that is harming you more than growing you, or that is stifling your growth in all areas of life, can no longer be. One of the hardest parts of a breakup is facing the reality that the relationship is over. The hurt that comes with that acknowledgement often makes us want to hate the person. How could they allow things to turn so sour, how could they not fight for you or change their ways? Believe it or not both partners typically play a part in some way in the relationships demise. This next line may make you want to close the book, but I am going to say it anyway. In your healing journey, you cannot afford the mental space it takes to hold anger in your heart or mind towards your ex. Go read that again. I wanted to be so angry, I wanted to cause physical and mental harm to my ex, because I couldn't imagine how I could be so horrible for him to not fight for us. I quickly had to learn to take the total blame off of him and look at the ways I neglected him. At one point in our marriage, work had become my partner, I will leave you to imagine what that did for my relationship. I also had to learn to give grace over anger. Trust me, family and friends wanted me to respond in a less gracious way, but along the journey I received so many confirmations from God that I was doing the right thing in offering grace. The most powerful part of the grace was the freedom it gave me. So now that you got the tea of my life, are you able to be honest with yourself?

Reflect on and answer the questions below:

- Is it really over?
- Why does this relationship need to be over for you?
- Where does it hurt?
- What is hard for you to fathom right now?
- What part did you play in the demise of your relationship (even if your part was getting in a relationship, you knew you should not have been in!)

_____

_____

_____

_____

_____

Reflections

_____

_____

_____

_____

_____

_____

_____

_____

Directions:

Take 10–15 minutes to write a letter to yourself acknowledging the end of the relationship. Express your feelings—whether it's sadness, relief, anger, or confusion—without judgment. Then, list three things you learned from the relationship and three ways you will focus on your healing moving forward. End the letter with words of encouragement to remind yourself that growth comes from endings.

Dear Self.....

_____

_____

_____

_____

_____

_____

_____

_____

_____

_____

_____

_____

_____

_____

_____

_____

_____

_____

_____

_____

_____

_____

_____

_____

_____

Dear Self.....

_____

_____

_____

_____

_____

_____

_____

_____

_____

_____

_____

_____

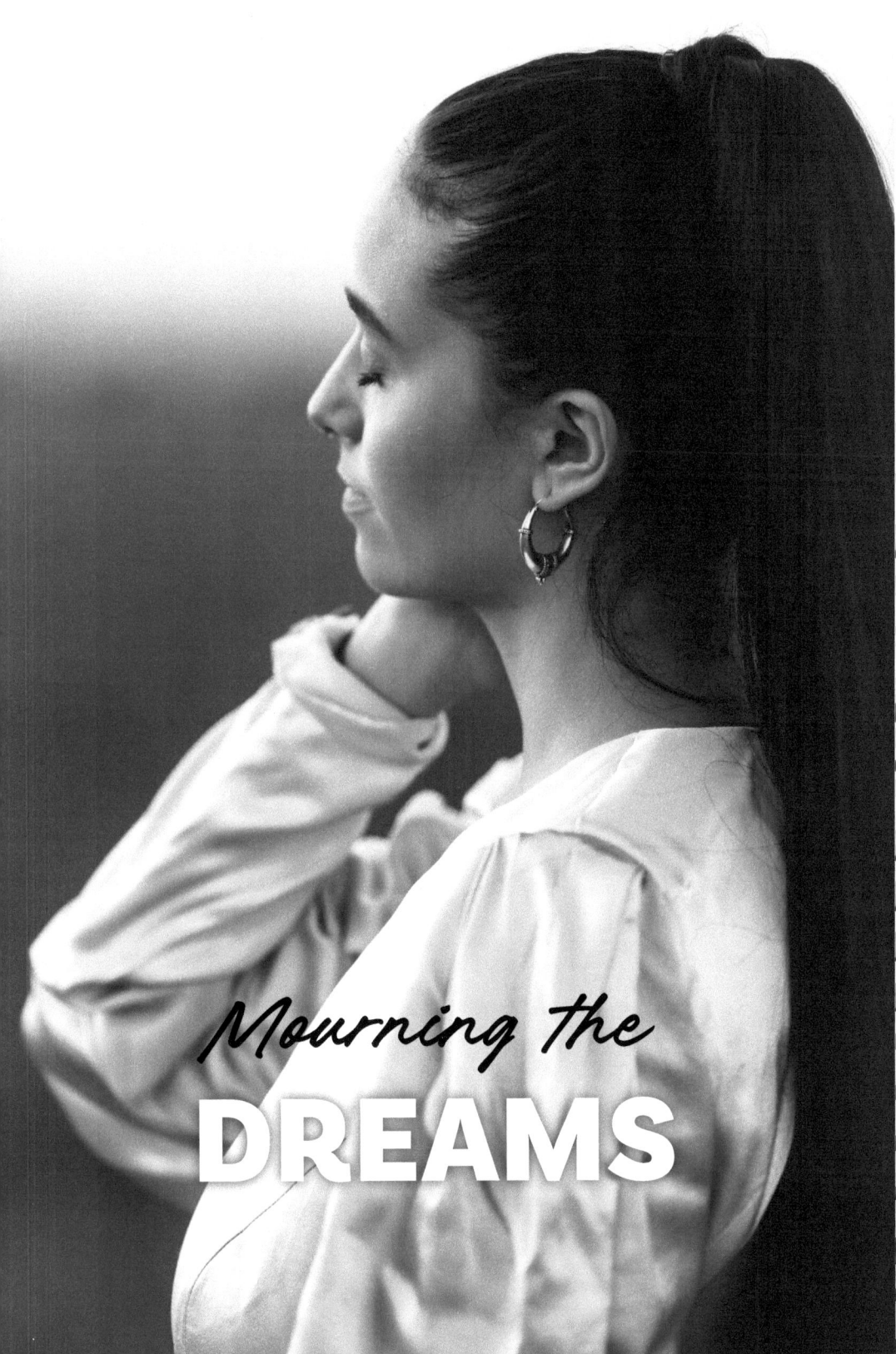

Mourning the

DREAMS

Mourning the Dreams

I am almost sure that at some point, you sat down with your partner and discussed the endless things you wanted to do together. Get married, maybe have children, buy a home, save money, vacation to that magical place you saw on social media. A lot of times when breaking up, we do not consider all the aspects of the relationship we are mourning. Not only is there the grief of losing the person including their mental and physical presence. We also mourn the safety they possibly provided, down to the closeness to their extended family including holiday get togethers.

There are so many adjustments that must occur, often leaving an empty void internally. For me it was the safety, the having someone consistently in the home with me, the comfort. So how do you find this peace again, how do you grieve in a manner that promotes self-growth. First, I implore that you do just that, grieve, allow your heart to cry out. Acknowledge every aspect that you will miss, that you are mourning, that you may be downright angry about losing. Sit in it, write it down, let your mind wander to what it could have been and then acknowledge that it will no longer be. You may not be to a space where you can reframe and create new dreams for yourself, we will get there. For now, we grieve while also loving on ourselves.

- What dreams are you mourning?
- Where do you feel the pain?
- What hope do you will for yourself today?
- What can you do to take care of yourself in the grief?

Set aside 15–20 minutes to create a 'Goodbye Ritual' to honor both the relationship and the dreams you had for its future. This could include writing a letter to the relationship expressing gratitude for the good moments, acknowledging the pain of letting go, and releasing any lingering hopes that no longer serve you. Afterward, choose a symbolic action, like tearing up the letter, burning it safely, or placing it in a box to store away, signifying your readiness to grieve, release, and begin healing.

_____

_____

_____

_____

_____

_____

_____

_____

_____

Reflections

_____

_____

_____

_____

_____

_____

_____

_____

_____

_____

_____

_____

_____

_____

_____

_____

_____

_____

_____

_____

_____

_____

_____

_____

_____

Reflections

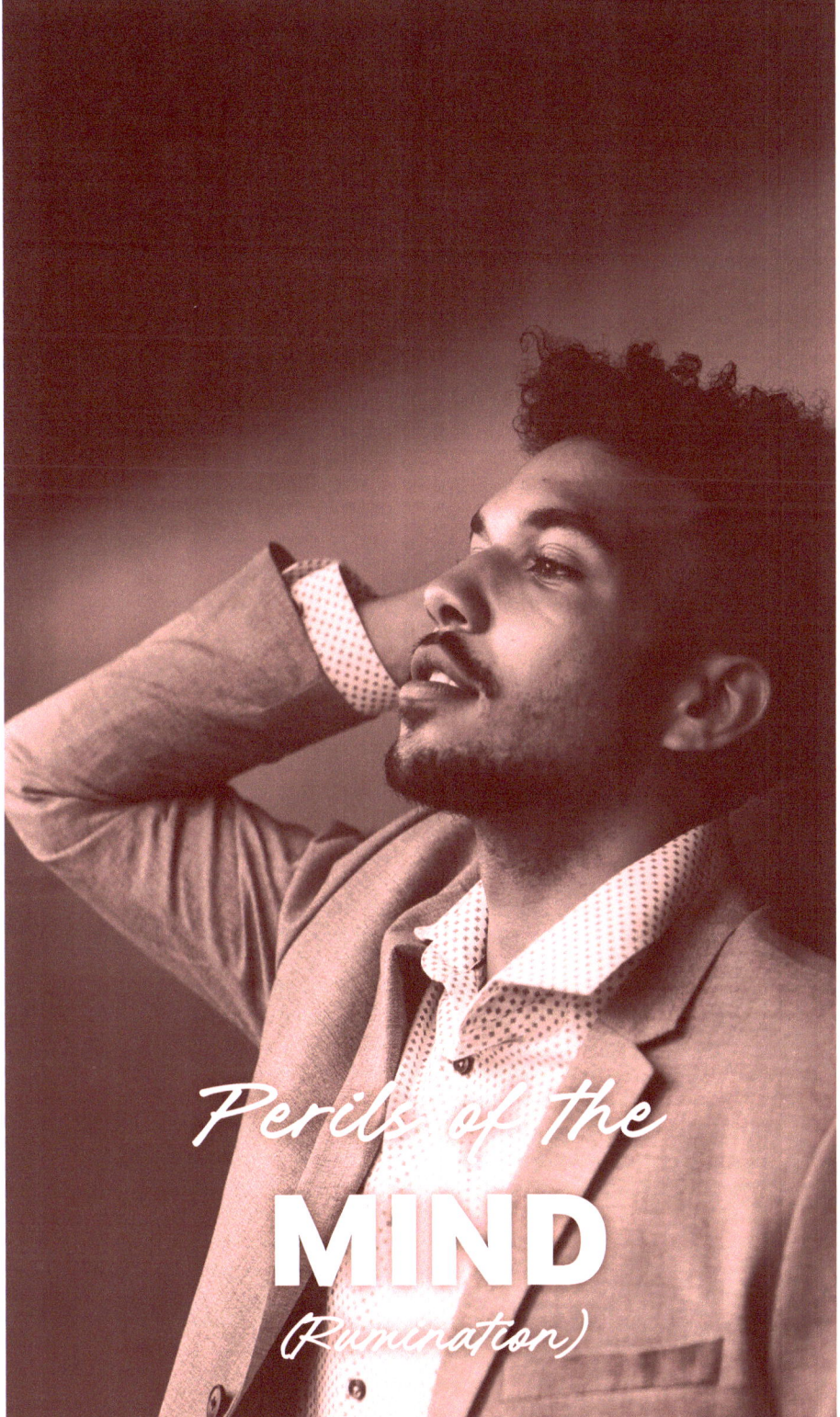

Perils of the

MIND

(Rumination)

Perils of the Mind

Look at you! Pushing through. You should be so proud of yourself, committing to this healing journey. So, let's talk about the perils (dangers) of the mind. I am going to take a wild guess that your mind has not been on your side since the breakup. I remember sitting in front of the television, but not being able to watch the show because my mind was going to every negative scenario it could think of. Did my partner give up because there was someone else? Was I not good enough? They were probably lying when......ahhhhhh! Your mind will ruminate, which means replay actual narratives and false ones.

The issue is, this will increase anxiety, anger, and overall is not a positive path towards your healing. If you recall, I am a trained mental health therapist, and there is a technique we use called thought stopping. This strategy involves blocking and replacing unwanted, distressing thoughts. In the previous pages, you already identified all the areas of the relationship that you are mourning. Therefore, we do not need to keep replaying them, we need to begin healing them. Well, how do I do that LaVante'? Great question!

The key is we want you to notice how often you are having these thoughts and distract you from them. These moments may also occur when a situation, smell, or place is a trigger for you. Therefore, using this thought stopping technique brings all of this to your awareness, and we want you totally aware. Bear in mind, we are not suppressing the thought, we are noticing it, stopping it, and replacing it with a positive one. Also, important to note is that I am a true believer in the power of mental health therapy. It is in those sessions that you can further process those thoughts.

For this book, we want to ensure that you can function on the job, with friends, and family in your daily life.

Here is the technique:

1. **Stop the thought:** Tell yourself stop, snap your finger, or write a check mark on a piece of paper to symbolize the thought has come again. You can even envision having a box with a lid that you place the thought in, put the lid on it to work through later.
2. **Notice the thought:** Remember, suppression is not the goal. Acknowledge that it exists without dwelling on it.
3. **Replace the thought:** Now the key is, you have to remember who you truly are! That you were made in His image! That you are unstoppable and that this too shall pass! Heck when I was in the brunt of my breakup, it felt like crawling out of an endless dark hole, but look at me now, shining in the light! Replace the thought with something more helpful, this can be a self-affirmation (you can also reference the "Who Am I?" section of this book.) You can also develop a mantra that helps you feel optimistic and focused.

At the time of my breakup, I found it impossible to believe positive things about myself, so I said this mantra to myself that I would say to my son, until I could believe it! "I am strong, I am brave, I am intelligent, I am unstoppable, I am LaVante'!" Feel free to borrow it if it speaks to you!

- What thoughts continue to ruminate through your mind?
- Which thought stopping technique do you feel could be helpful? (Reference #1 above)
- Who are you! Write 5 breathtaking affirmations about yourself, even if you do not believe them yet.

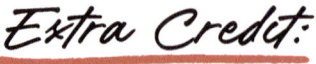

Extra Credit:

Develop a mantra for yourself.

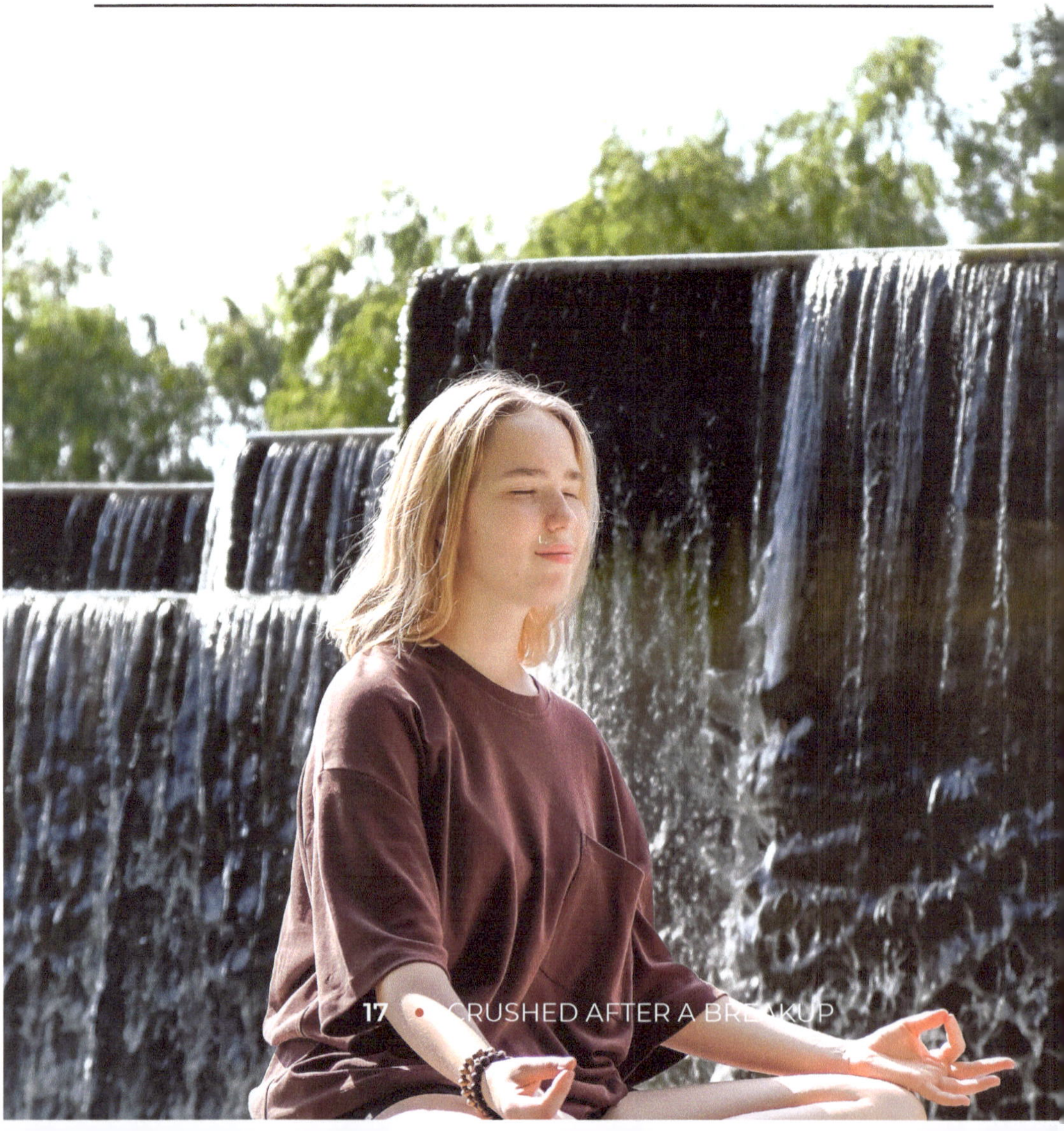

_____

_____

_____

_____

Reflections

_____

_____

_____

_____

_____

_____

_____

_____

_____

_____

_____

_____

Reflections

_____

_____

_____

_____

_____

_____

_____

_____

_____

_____

_____

_____

_____

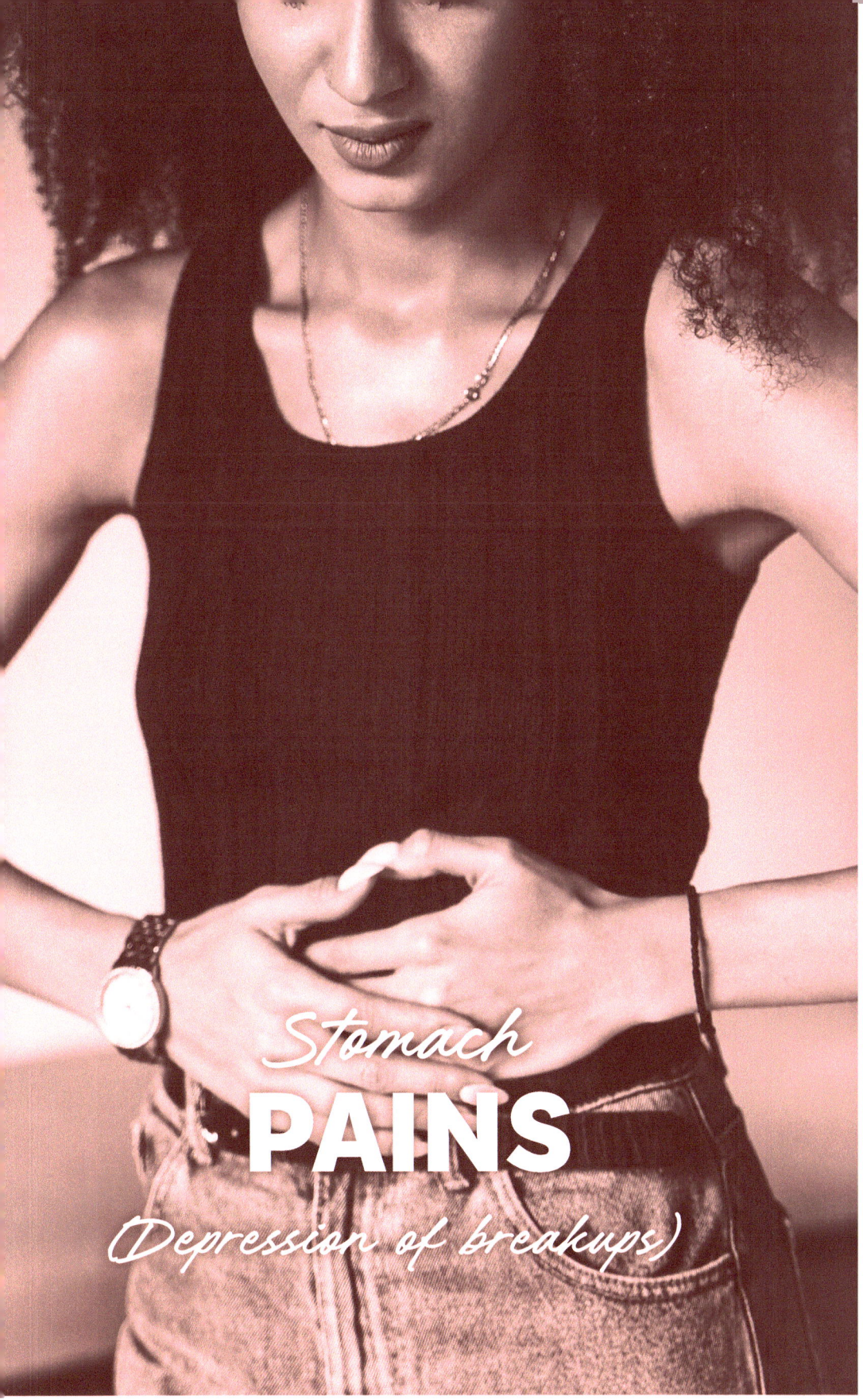

Stomach
PAINS
(Depression of breakups)

Stomach Pains

I remember the day I realized my marriage was over. I couldn't eat and the only time the anxious stomach pains ended was during the few hours of sleep that I could get. The challenging part of my anxiety and depression at the time due to the breakup was that I was also in the period after childbirth in which women can experience post-partum depression. Yes, this was all happening three months after giving birth to my son. If you read that and felt a sense of "Oh, heck no!" remember, grace.

When we face anxiety and depression, we must first acknowledge the physical pains we feel. This may be an increase in headaches, sleepiness, stomach pains, the body has an interesting way of processing emotional hurt. We then must truly ask ourselves what is challenging for me right now?

Being around friends and family, showering, eating, drinking water, going outside, doing work, you name it. If any of these things are occurring, we must not ignore them. You have to push yourself to do the opposite, do them!

Showers became my solace, the warm water while listening to an encouraging sermon gave me the temporary peace I needed to breathe. I also made my closest friends and family aware of what was going on and boy did they show up.

I was intentional to step outside if even for a moment and get fresh air or sit under the stars and pray. I was in such a vulnerable space for my life to be unraveling before my eyes. But remember that choice, I made the choice that even if I could not see why I was going through it, I would live. I deserved to, and my son did as well.

- How is your body responding physically to your breakup?
- Describe what else is going on in your life that is adding to the challenge of the breakup.
- In what way can you give grace today?
- What activity do you need to start again today?

1. Am I experiencing any changes in my sleep patterns, such as difficulty falling asleep, staying asleep, or oversleeping?
2. Have I noticed any changes in my appetite or eating habits, such as loss of appetite, overeating, or craving certain foods?
3. Do I feel any physical tension or discomfort, such as headaches, muscle pain, or a tight feeling in my chest?
4. Am I experiencing any changes in my energy levels, such as feeling constantly fatigued or unusually restless?
5. Have I noticed any changes in my exercise or physical activity levels, either avoiding it or using it as a coping mechanism?
6. Am I experiencing any digestive issues, such as stomach aches, nausea, or other gastrointestinal disturbances?

Exercise:

Take 10–15 minutes to sit quietly and do a full body scan. Close your eyes, take deep breaths, and notice any areas of tension, heaviness, or discomfort in your body. Gently place your hand on the area where you feel the most pain and acknowledge it without judgment. Journal about what sensations you noticed and what emotions might be connected to them. End with a grounding activity, such as stretching, yoga, or a short walk, to help release stored tension.

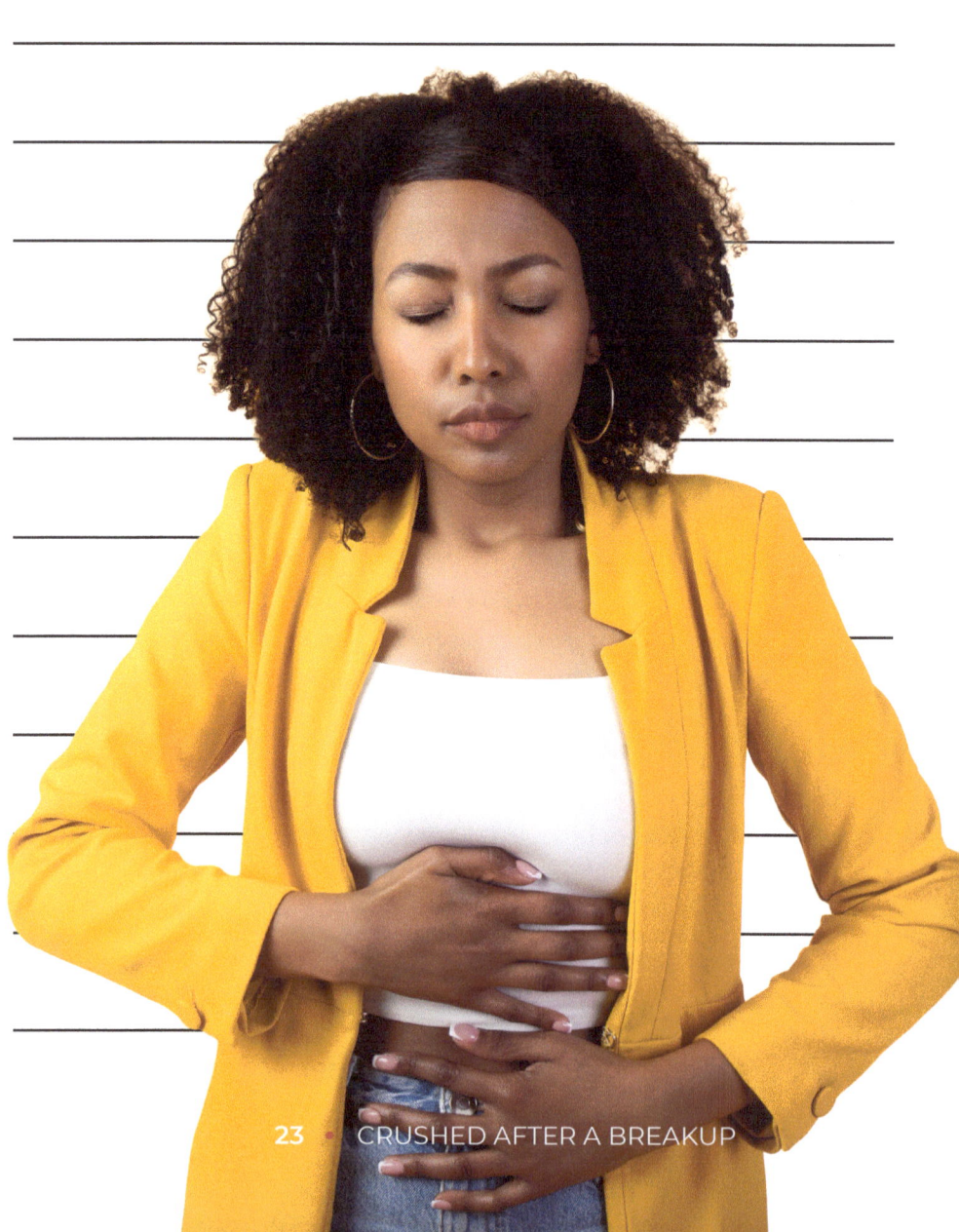

Reflections

_____

_____

_____

_____

_____

_____

_____

_____

_____

_____

_____

_____

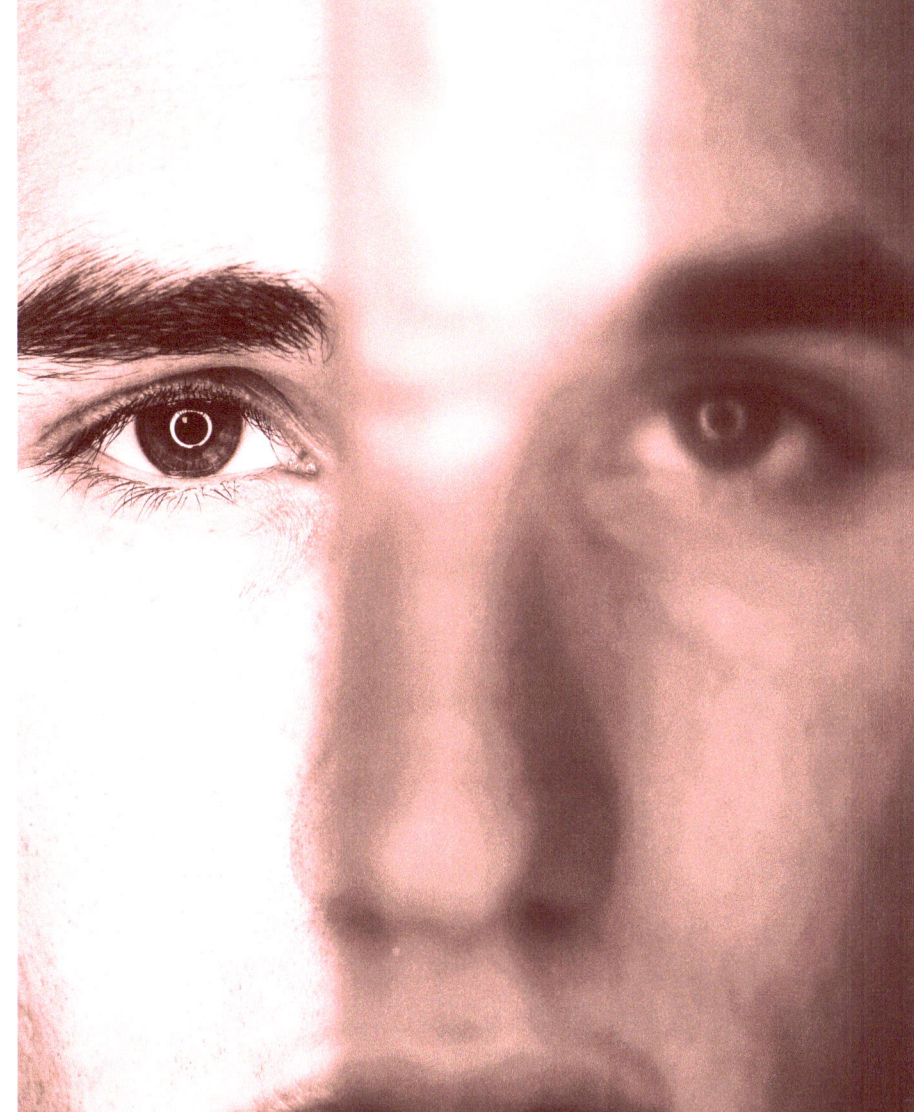

The Truth of the

MATTER

(Was this healthy for you?)

The Truth of the Matter

Still pushing I see! You are amazing! Question; have you looked back yet and considered if your ex was actually a good partner for you? Reminder, I am not saying that they are a bad person, unless your ex truly needed to do their own healing work. I am saying when you think of your values, when you think of your peace and happiness and dreams, did your ex truly fit the bill? We also must consider were you the best version of your self for your ex?

Remember that I stated I was able to look at my shortcomings as well, my controlling ways that were not healthy for a relationship. A lot of times we hold onto a sort of fantasy of what the relationship was or could have been. The hopes we had versus the truth of the two people that were showing up in the relationship.

So when you sit and consider this, what say ye?

1. Did my ex support my personal growth and encourage me to pursue my goals and dreams?
2. Did I feel valued and respected in the relationship, or did I often feel criticized or undermined?
3. Was there a healthy balance of give and take, or did I feel like I was constantly giving more than I received?
4. Did my ex communicate openly and honestly, or were there frequent misunderstandings and secrets?
5. How did my ex handle conflicts—were they resolved constructively, or did they often lead to more harm and resentment?
6. Reflecting on the relationship, did I feel happier and more confident with my ex, or did I often feel anxious, sad, or unworthy?

Reflections

_____

_____

_____

_____

_____

_____

_____

_____

_____

_____

_____

Reflections

_____

_____

_____

_____

_____

_____

_____

_____

_____

_____

_____

_____

_____

Make a list of the qualities and values that are most important to you in a healthy relationship. Then, create two columns—one for what your ex-partner brought to the relationship and another for what was missing or misaligned. Reflect on whether their actions and behaviors truly supported your emotional, mental, and physical well-being. Journal about any patterns you notice and how this insight can guide you in future relationships.

Important qualities for a healthy relationship:

_____

_____

_____

_____

_____

_____

_____

_____

_____

Good Qualities:

_____

_____

_____

_____

_____

_____

_____

_____

_____

_____

_____

Missing Qualities:

_____

_____

_____

_____

_____

_____

_____

_____

_____

_____

_____

Grace over anger and
REVENGE

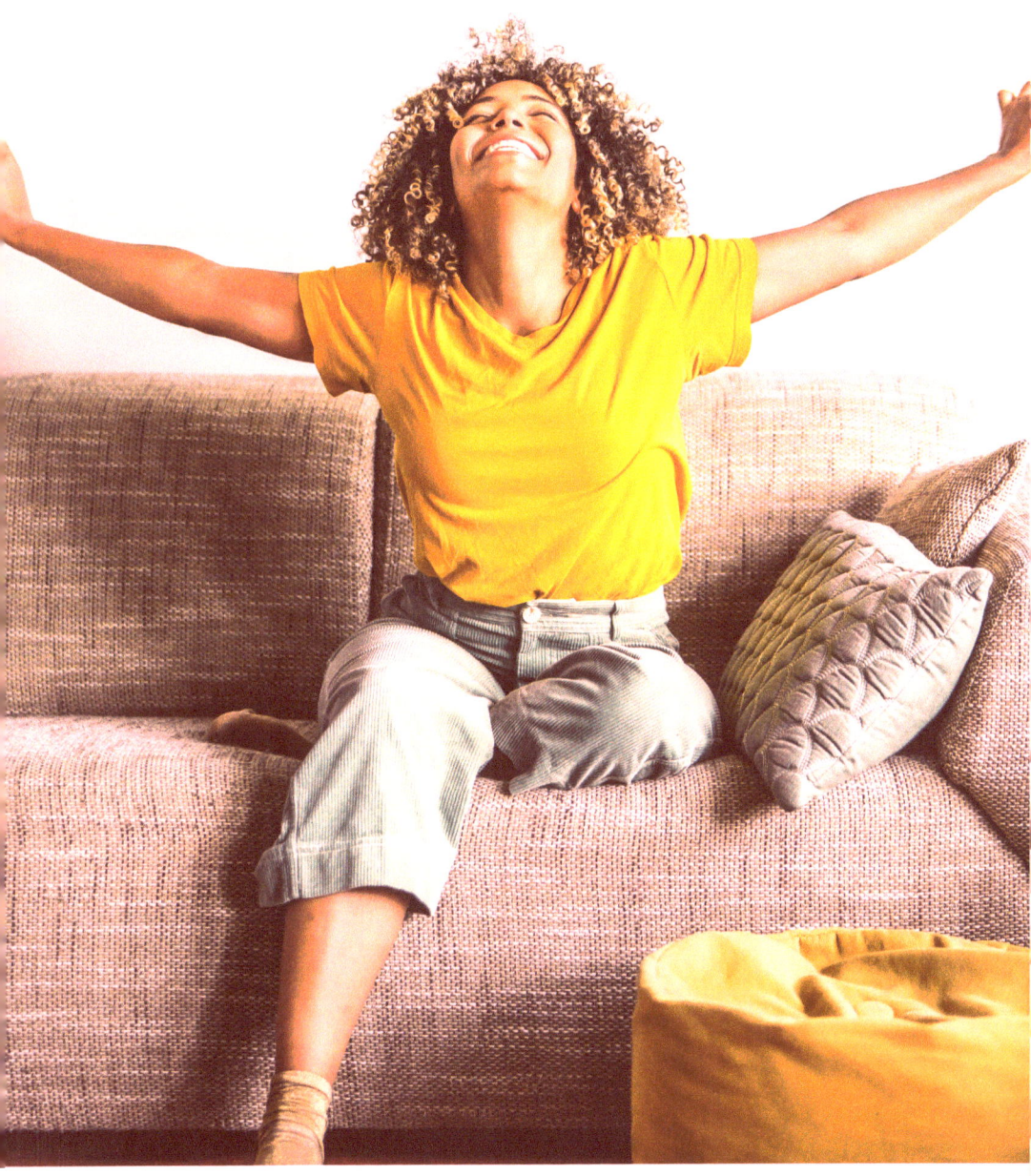

Grace Over Anger and Revenge

In my line of work as a mental health therapist, I work with a lot of people processing a breakup. It is very interesting how creative the mind can get when it is angry and wanting to "get back" at the person who hurt you. I decided very early on that anger and revenge would not be the actions I took in my breakup.

My spirituality called me to take a higher ground, my inner person who I strive to be called me higher, and most importantly my son. I had seen too often how quarreling parents effected the children and I refused for that to be my story.

Now that didn't mean I didn't get angry and it sure didn't mean my mind didn't think of revenge. (I am chuckling as I write this.) What it meant was when I was angry, I talked it out with my own therapists and friends, or took a walk and listened to my gospel music. It also didn't mean that I was a push over, I created my boundaries, I still let my ex-partner know how I felt, and most of all I gave grace. I would describe grace as a sort of pass. As in you have stomped over my heart, but I am going to forgive you and let you go. I am going to be kind even though you deserve my wrath! Am I making sense, just like Michelle Obama said, "when they go low, we go high!"

1. What specific actions or behaviors from my ex are fueling my feelings of anger and desire for revenge?
2. How might seeking revenge impact my own emotional well-being and personal growth in the long run?
3. Can I identify any underlying emotions, such as hurt or betrayal, that are contributing to my desire for revenge?
4. What positive outcomes could come from choosing to give grace and forgiveness, both for myself and for my future relationships?
5. How would I feel if I were to respond with kindness and understanding instead of anger—would it bring me more peace

and closure?

6. What steps can I take to channel my anger into constructive activities that promote healing and self-improvement, rather than focusing on revenge?

Set aside 15–20 minutes to release your anger in a healthy way. Try a physical activity like going for a run, hitting a punching bag, or dancing to high-energy music. If you prefer a creative outlet, write an uncensored letter to your ex (you don't have to send it) or paint or draw what your anger feels like. Afterward, take a few deep breaths and reflect on how releasing that energy made you feel. Journal about any remaining emotions and what you need to continue letting go.

_____

_____

_____

_____

_____

_____

_____

_____

Reflections

_____

_____

_____

_____

_____

_____

_____

_____

_____

_____

_____

_____

Reflections

_____

_____

_____

_____

_____

_____

_____

_____

_____

_____

_____

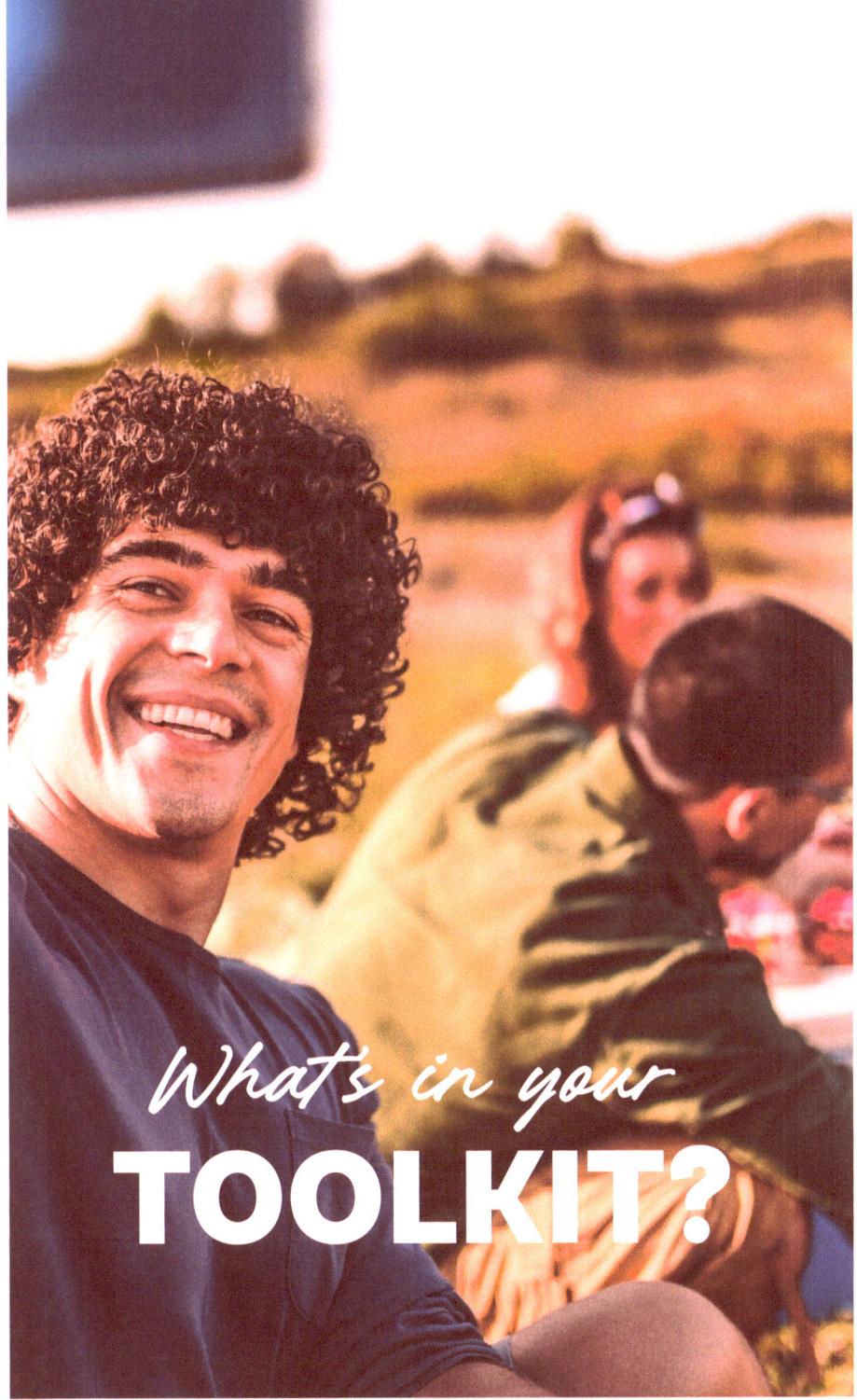

What's in your
TOOLKIT?

What's in your Toolkit?

When challenging emotions are built up inside, we need a way to release them. A lot of time we turn to vices that may not serve us the way we need, because they mask versus address the issue. We may be urged to drink alcohol to mask the pain or find ways to avoid it. If you have found yourself in a space of avoidance, I challenge you to consider a different approach.

Other approaches could be meeting with a trained therapist to talk out your problems, yoga, breathwork, working out, journaling, anything that releases the feelings versus stuffing them. Walking at the riverfront became my best friend, I escaped into nature, prayed, cried, whatever I need in the moment. Those painful moments would quickly turn into peace when I could encourage myself to know that this was not the end of my journey and one day I would be in a healthy and loving relationship.

1. Am I engaging in any behaviors that I know are harmful or self-destructive, such as excessive drinking, drug use, or self-isolation?
2. How am I managing my emotions—am I expressing them in healthy ways, such as talking to a friend or therapist, or am I bottling them up or lashing out at others?
3. Am I taking care of my physical health by maintaining a balanced diet, getting regular exercise, and ensuring adequate sleep, or am I neglecting these aspects of my well-being?
4. Have I established any new routines or activities that bring me joy and relaxation, such as hobbies, mindfulness practices, or social engagements, or am I avoiding these positive outlets?
5. Am I allowing myself to process my feelings at my own pace, or am I trying to rush through the healing process by seeking distractions or rebound relationships?
6. How often am I reflecting on my own needs and boundaries, and am I making decisions that prioritize my long-term emotional health over short-term comfort or escape?

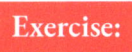

Create a 'Coping Skills Treasure Box':

1. **Find a Box or Container:** Pick something fun, like a colorful box, a mason jar, or even a small suitcase. Decorate it with stickers, quotes, or drawings that inspire positivity.
2. **Gather Your Tools:** Fill the box with items that soothe, distract, or uplift you. Some ideas:
    • **Sensory Items:** Stress balls, scented candles, or fidget toys.
    • **Creative Tools:** Coloring books, journals, or sketchpads.
    • **Comfort Items:** Photos, a favorite book, or a soft blanket.
    • **Inspirational Notes:** Write affirmations, motivational quotes, or letters to your future self.
    • **Distraction Activities:** Puzzle books, cards, or playlists with uplifting music.
3. **Try One New Coping Skill This Week:** Pick something you've never tried before, like guided meditation, yoga, or learning a dance routine from a video. Write down how it made you feel and whether you'd add it to your toolkit.
4. **Schedule Check-Ins:** Each week, revisit your box and add new tools or replace ones that no longer serve you.

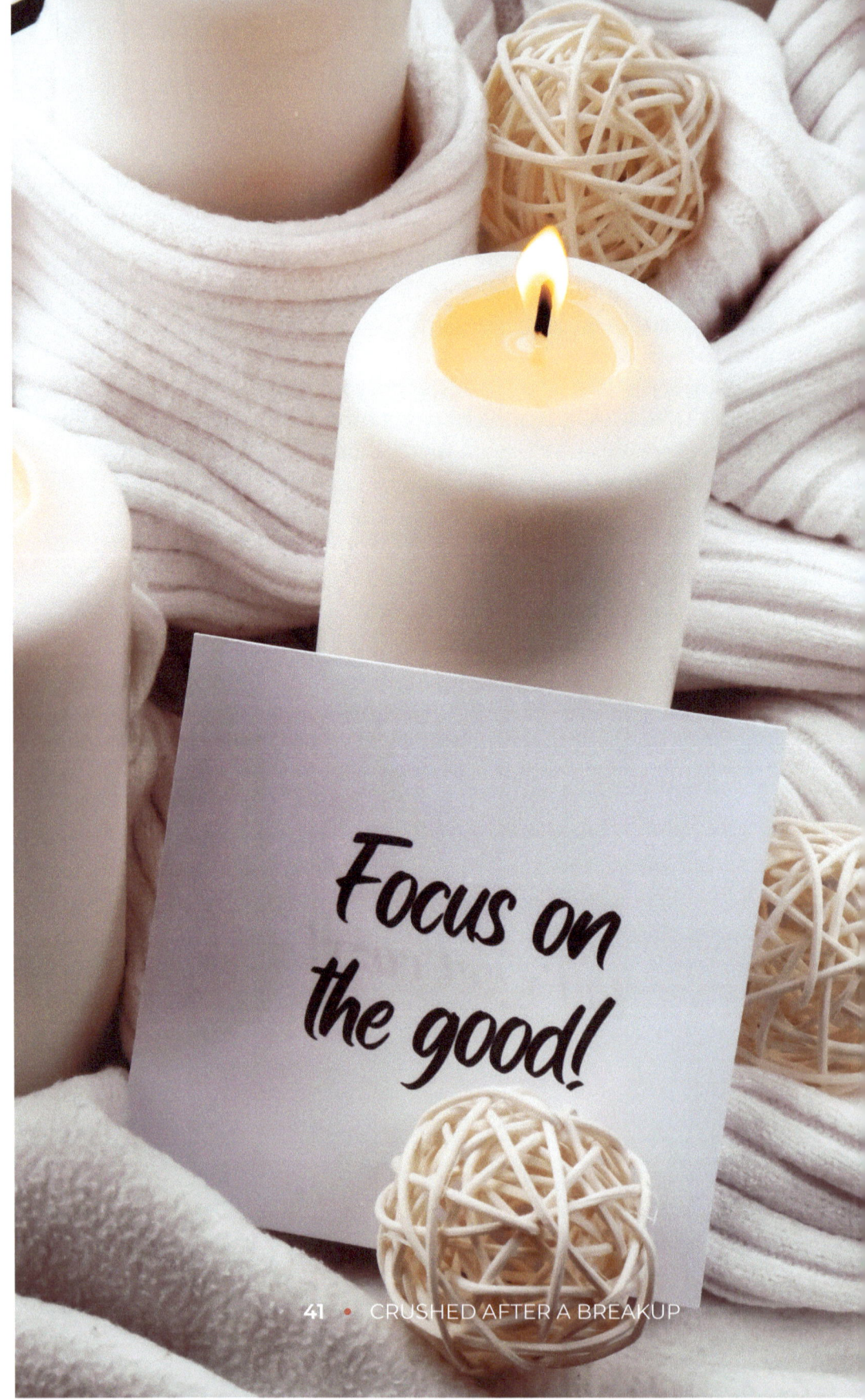

Focus on
the good!

Reflections

_____

_____

_____

_____

_____

_____

_____

_____

_____

_____

_____

_____

Reflections

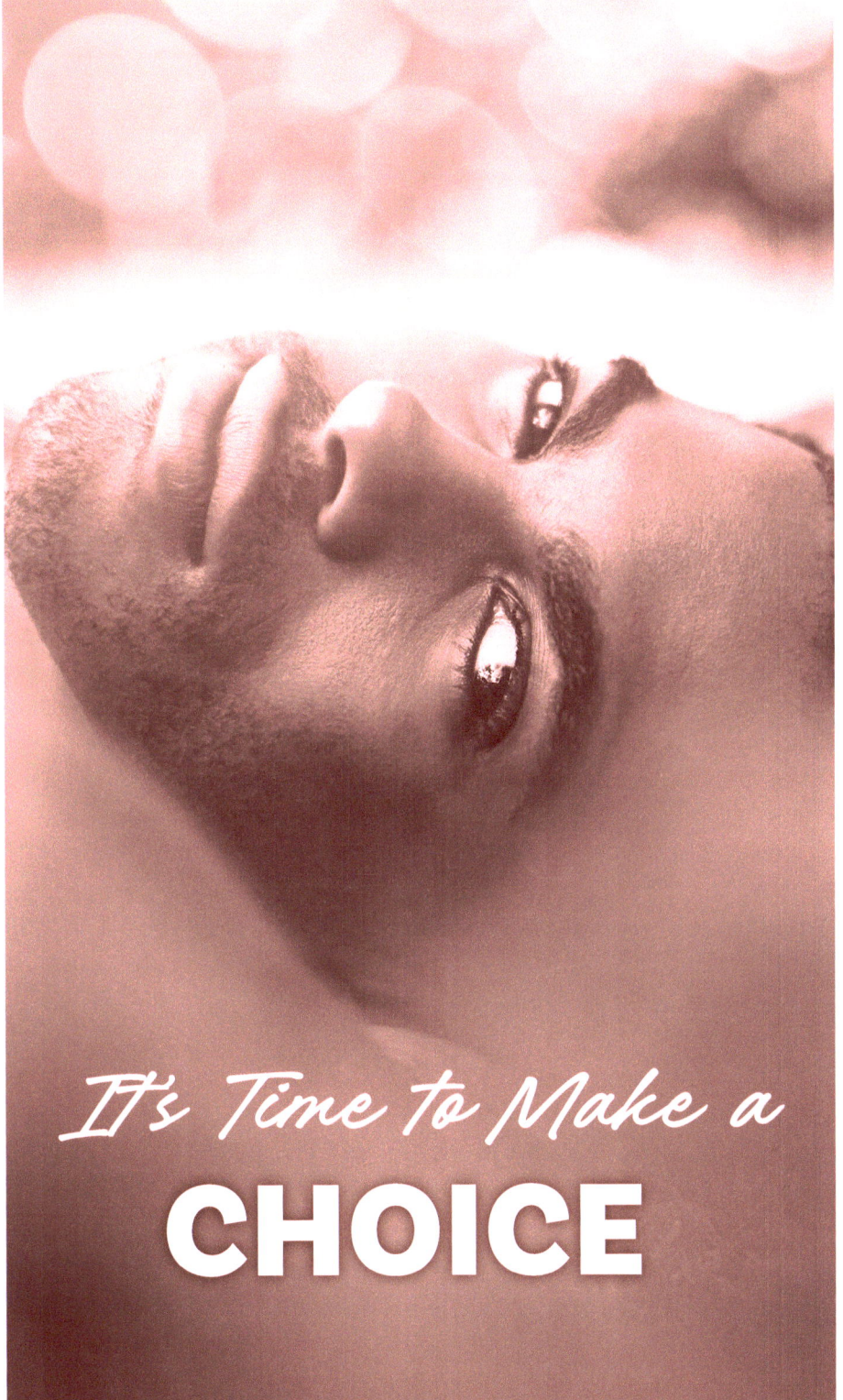

It's Time to Make a Choice

Life and death are in the power of the tongue. That sentence didn't hit me until it did. I had a choice to make, be down in the dumps, depressed, give up, or overcome. I thought of all the reasons I couldn't give up, I had a son to care for, a house to take care of, a business to manage, youth to inspire, and clients to help. I had a choice; you have a choice.

The first couple of days, I was so hurt and anxious, I couldn't eat, sleep well, or find the motivation to complete needed tasks. I still recall sitting on the couch and saying out loud, "God, help me!" Now remember I am telling you who helped me, you have a choice to make. A choice for yourself, will you let this breakup take you down, or will you soar above and come out better than before?

1. What goals and dreams did I have before this relationship, and how can I refocus on them now to create a fulfilling future?
2. In what ways can I use this breakup as an opportunity for personal growth and self-discovery?
3. What positive changes and new opportunities could arise from pressing forward and not giving up on myself and my happiness?
4. How can I reframe my mindset to view this breakup as a stepping stone rather than a setback?
5. What support systems (friends, family, therapists) can I lean on to help me navigate this challenging time and encourage me to keep moving forward?
6. What specific steps can I take today to begin rebuilding my life and fostering resilience in the face of this adversity?

Reflections

_____

_____

_____

_____

_____

_____

_____

_____

_____

_____

_____

_____

Reflections

_____

_____

_____

_____

_____

_____

_____

_____

_____

_____

_____

_____

_____

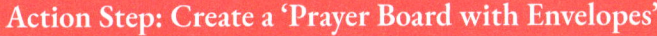

Supplies Needed:

- Poster board or corkboard
- 6 envelopes
- Markers, pens, stickers, and decorations
- Index cards or small pieces of paper
- Tape or push pins

Steps to Create Your Prayer Board:

1. **Label the Envelopes with Categories:**
   - **Gratitude** – Prayers of thankfulness and blessings already received.
   - **Healing** – Prayers for emotional, physical, and spiritual healing.
   - **Guidance** – Requests for clarity, wisdom, and direction in decision-making.
   - **Relationships** – Prayers for family, friends, and new or restored connections.
   - **Dreams & Goals** – Hopes and aspirations for the future.
   - **Prayers Answered** – Celebrate prayers that have been fulfilled.
2. **Attach the Envelopes to the Board:**
   - Tape or pin each envelope in an organized, visually appealing layout. Feel free to decorate with stickers, Bible verses, or affirmations.
3. **Fill the Envelopes:**
   - Write prayers on index cards or small slips of paper and place them into the appropriate envelopes.
   - Be specific and heartfelt, trusting in the process.

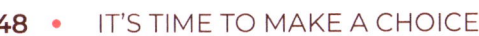

4. **Daily or Weekly Prayer Time:**
   - Set aside time to review and pray over the cards in each envelope.
   - Add new prayers as needed.
5. **Celebrate Prayers Answered:**
   - Move any fulfilled prayers to the **'Prayers Answered'** envelope.
   - Reflect and give thanks for what has come to pass.
6. **Maintain and Reflect:**
   - Regularly review the board and update it with new prayers and goals.
   - Use this time as an opportunity to stay grounded in faith and gratitude.

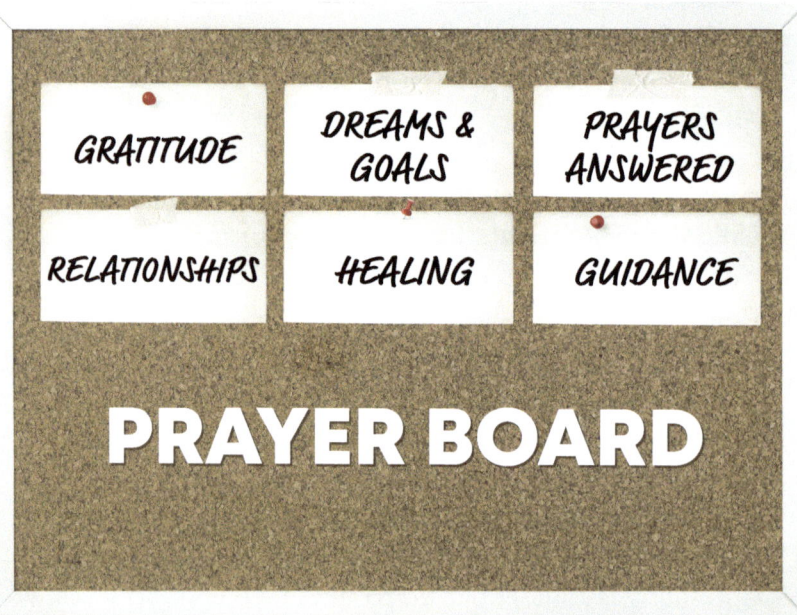

Optional Addition:

Include motivational quotes, scriptures, or pictures that remind you to trust the process and stay hopeful. This prayer board provides a visual reminder of faith, hope, and progress while encouraging reflection and gratitude!

When will the pain
END?

When Will The Pain End?

Is this a trick question? I am a few years out and moments of pain and mourning still pop up. Everyone's healing has a unique timeline. The pain and mourning after a breakup can vary significantly from person to person. We have to remember that many factors such as the length and depth of the relationship, the circumstances of the breakup, and individual coping mechanisms can influence that timeline.

Generally, it's normal for the intense feelings of grief and sadness to last several weeks to a few months. However, the process of healing and moving on can take longer, sometimes up to a year or more, as individuals work through their emotions and gradually rebuild their sense of self and normalcy. It's important to remember that healing is not linear, and giving oneself grace and patience during this period is crucial.

Seeking support from friends, family, or a therapist can also be beneficial in navigating the complex emotions that arise after a breakup. There goes that grace again, and now you are giving it to yourself.

1. Am I allowing myself to fully feel and express my emotions, understanding that it's okay to experience sadness, anger, and confusion during this time?
2. How can I practice self-compassion and be gentle with myself, recognizing that healing is a gradual process that cannot be rushed?
3. What small, nurturing activities can I incorporate into my daily routine to support my emotional well-being and promote self-care?
4. Am I being patient with myself and acknowledging that setbacks are a natural part of the healing journey?

5. How can I remind myself that it's okay to seek help and lean on my support network when I'm feeling overwhelmed or lonely?
6. In what ways can I celebrate the small victories and progress I make along the way, even if they seem minor in the grand scheme of my healing process?

Action Step:

1. **Schedule Time to Grieve:** Set aside 10–15 minutes each day to sit with your emotions. Write in a journal, cry, or listen to music that helps you process your feelings without judgment.
2. **Practice Self-Compassion:** Write down affirmations such as, *'Healing takes time, and I deserve to move through this at my own pace.'* Repeat these daily to counter the urge to rush.
3. **Focus on Small Wins:** Each day, write down one thing you did for yourself—whether it's getting out of bed, going for a walk, or reaching out to a friend. Celebrate these moments as progress.
4. **Ground Yourself in the Present:** Engage in mindfulness activities like deep breathing, yoga, or meditation to help you stay grounded and resist the urge to fast-forward through your healing process.

Reflections

_____

_____

_____

_____

_____

_____

_____

_____

_____

_____

_____

_____

Reflections

_____

_____

_____

_____

_____

_____

_____

_____

_____

_____

_____

_____

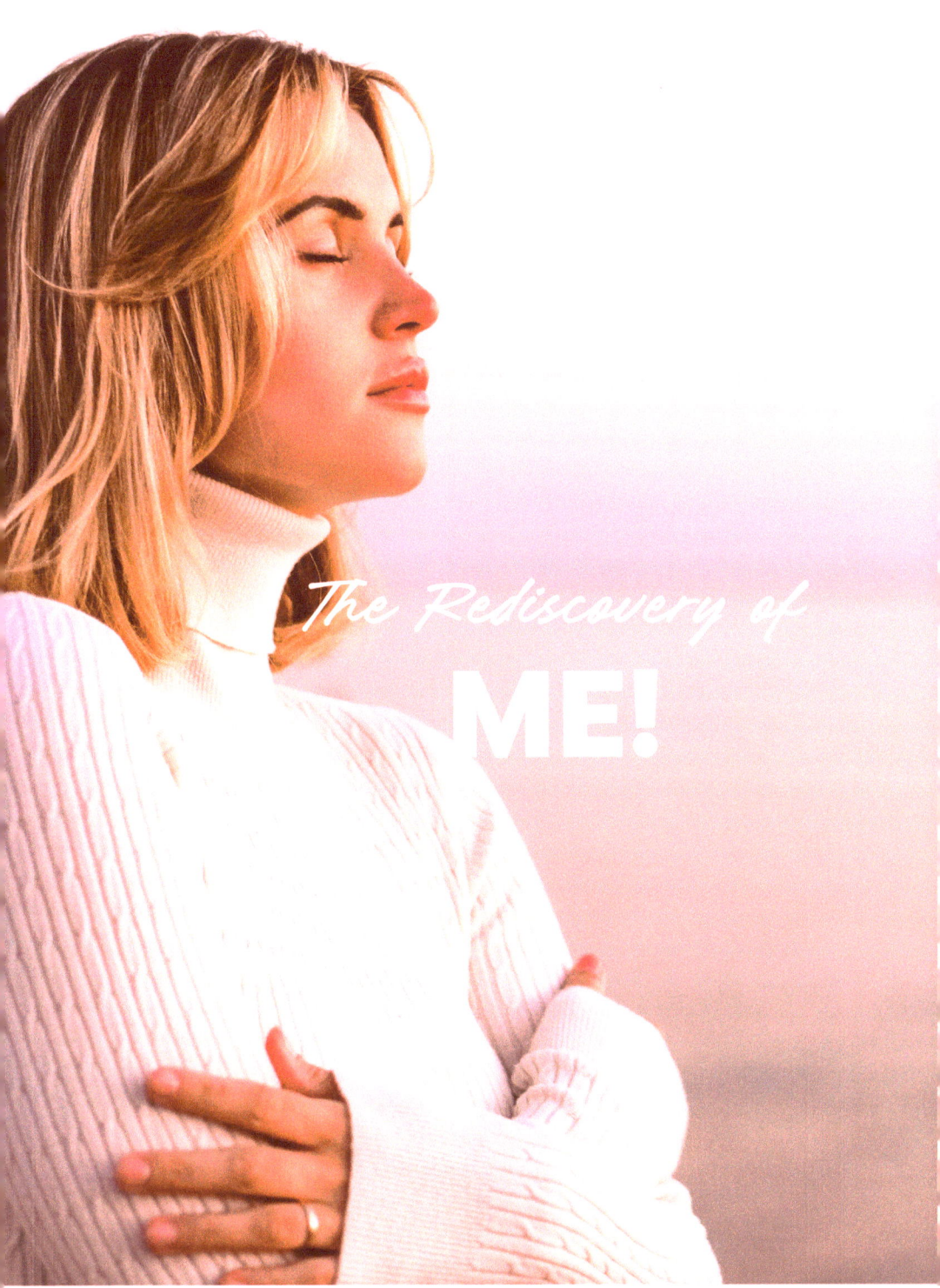

The Rediscovery of
ME!

The Rediscovery of Me!

I had been in my relationship for 8 years. Who the heck was I now that it was over?

Rediscovering yourself after a breakup is an empowering journey of self-exploration and growth. Take this time to reconnect with your passions, interests, and goals that may have been set aside during the relationship. Embrace new hobbies, revisit old ones, and allow yourself to try new experiences that spark joy and curiosity. Reflect on your strengths and achievements, and use this period to redefine your values and aspirations.

You are amazing, and sometimes during the hurtful journey, we forget that! I remember the day I became intentional and less predictable. I did not allow worries and lack to dictate my moves. I wanted to just be, to live, to take impromptu trips to the beach, mini weekends away, and take myself on dates.

1. What hobbies or activities did I enjoy before the relationship that I might want to revisit or explore further now?
2. What new experiences or interests have I always wanted to try but never had the chance to pursue?
3. What personal strengths and qualities have I discovered or reinforced during this challenging time?
4. How can I reconnect with my goals and dreams, and what steps can I take to start working towards them again?
5. Who are the supportive people in my life that I can lean on for encouragement and inspiration as I rediscover myself?
6. What self-care practices can I incorporate into my daily routine to nurture my emotional and physical well-being during this period of self-discovery?

"Create a 'Who Am I Now?' Journal!"

1. **Reflect on Your Core Values:** Write down 5-10 values that feel most important to you right now (e.g., honesty, growth, independence, love). Reflect on how these values may have shifted after your breakup.
2. **Explore Your Beliefs:** Journal about what you now believe about love, relationships, and yourself. Challenge any limiting beliefs and rewrite them into empowering ones.
3. **Clarify Your Desires:** Write out what you truly want in this new season of life—emotionally, spiritually, and physically. Be bold and specific.
4. **Take One Action:** Pick one small activity this week that aligns with your new values or desires—whether it's signing up for a class, volunteering, or spending time in nature—and commit to it.

Bonus: Revisit this journal weekly to track your growth and refine your vision as you continue discovering who you are becoming.

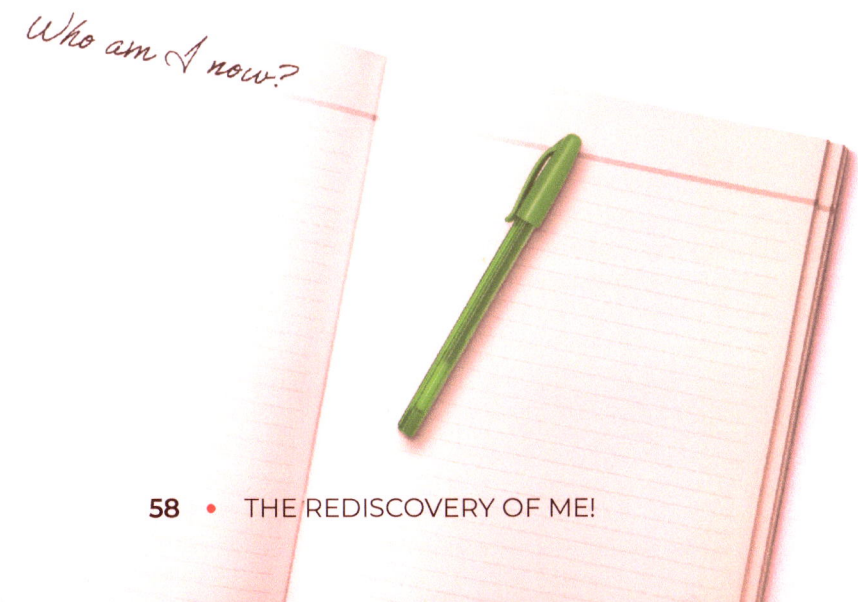

Reflections

_____

_____

_____

_____

_____

_____

_____

_____

_____

_____

_____

_____

_____

Reflections

_____

_____

_____

_____

_____

_____

_____

_____

_____

_____

_____

_____

Reflections

_____

_____

_____

_____

_____

_____

_____

_____

_____

_____

_____

_____

_____

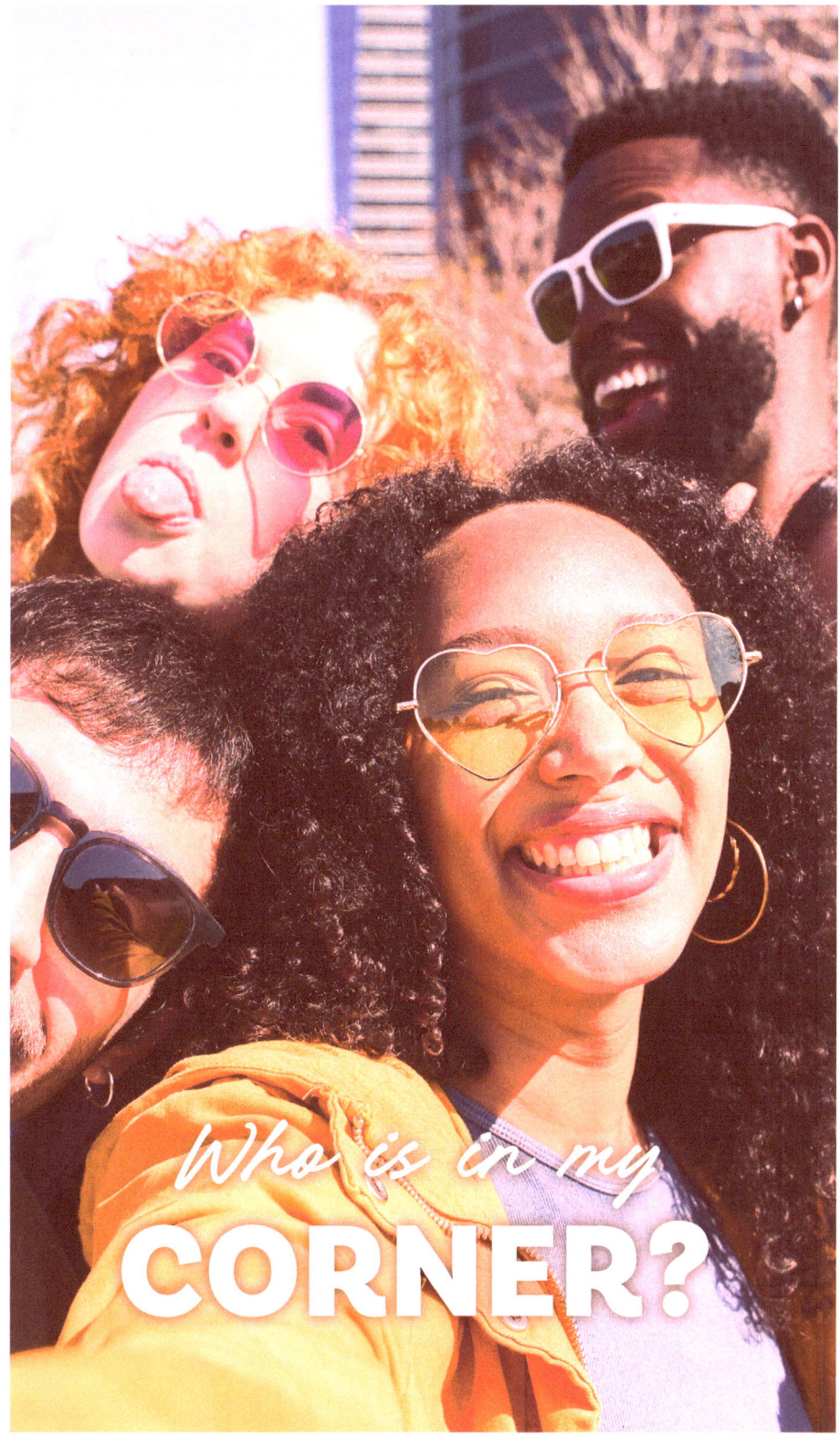

Who is in my
CORNER?

Who is in My Corner?

Countless times in my therapy sessions with clients I discuss not abandoning your village. Typically, in our worst moments we go into a shell of isolation not wanting to experience the shame of telling others how much pain we are in regarding relationship woes.

They won't understand, they are tired of hearing my stories, they will judge me. Well, if your village treats you like that, you need a new village! Now is the time more than ever to lean on your village and allow them to show up for you, just as you have them.

1. **Reflection on Support System:**
   - Who is currently part of your "village"?
   - How have they shown up for you in the past during difficult times?
2. **Self-Assessment of Isolation:**
   - When faced with challenges, do you tend to isolate yourself? Why or why not?
   - What emotions come up for you when you think about reaching out for help?
3. **Evaluating Your Village:**
   - Do you feel supported, understood, and accepted by your current village? Why or why not?
   - Are there people in your life who make you feel judged or unheard? How does that impact your willingness to share with them?
4. **Building a Better Village:**
   - If you feel your current village is lacking support, what qualities would you look for in a healthier support system?
   - What steps can you take to strengthen your village or build new connections?

5. **Giving and Receiving Support:**
   - How have you shown up for others in your village during their struggles?
   - How do you feel about allowing others to show up for you in return?
6. **Overcoming Shame and Fear:**
   - What fears or insecurities hold you back from sharing your struggles with others?
   - How can you challenge these thoughts and remind yourself of the value of connection?

This week, identify one trusted person in your village and reach out to them. Share something that's been on your mind—big or small—and allow yourself to be open to their support. Then, reflect on how it felt to lean on your village and write about it in your journal.

_____

_____

_____

_____

_____

_____

_____

Reflections

_____

_____

_____

_____

_____

_____

_____

_____

_____

_____

_____

_____

Reflections

_____

_____

_____

_____

_____

_____

_____

_____

_____

_____

_____

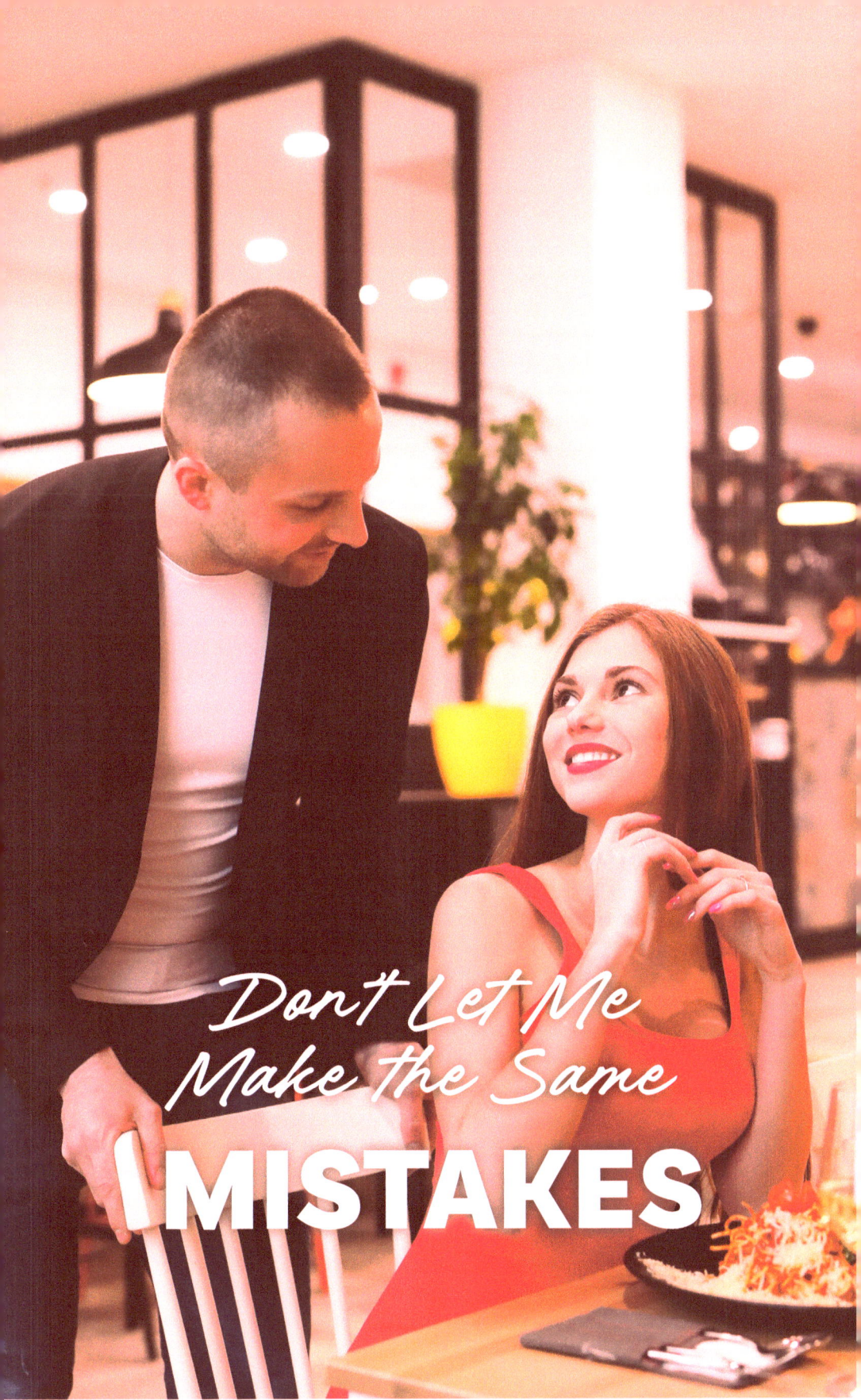

Don't Let Me Make the Same **MISTAKES**

Don't Let Me Make the Same Mistakes

One of the scariest and anxiety provoking parts is once you are healed and considering love again. Yes, although you have done great work, there is still work to be done. One thing we do not want to do is choose the wrong person again or be hurt again in similar ways.

A lot of times we have a type, or we choose people with not just similar physical characteristics but similar personalities, values, and beliefs. Therefore, this is where we want to take the time to recalibrate and consider what we do really want in a mate. More importantly, who God has made for us.

Now if you are anything like me, I have a list and a file saved on Instagram with videos that represent some of the characteristics I desire in a partner. We want to pay attention to how we are valued, how a partner shows up for us, learns and studies us, as well as prays for us, and that they have a solid relationship with God. I am not referring to the play one either, but the genuine relationship where you can see them seeking God.

Follow-Up Questions for Reflection:

1. **Personal Growth and Readiness:**
   - What fears or hesitations do I still have about opening my heart to love again?
   - What lessons have I learned from my past relationships that I want to carry forward?
2. **Defining Desires in a Partner:**
   - What qualities, values, and beliefs do I want in a future partner?
   - How do I want my future partner to show up for me emotionally, spiritually, and physically?
3. **Spiritual Alignment:**
   - How important is my partner's relationship with God to me?

- What does a healthy spiritual connection in a relationship look like to me?

4. **Patterns and Preferences:**
   - Have I noticed patterns in the types of people I've been drawn to in the past?
   - Are those patterns healthy or do they need to change?

Create Your Relationship Blueprint:

1. **List Your Non-Negotiables:** Write down the top 5 qualities or values that you cannot compromise in a partner (e.g., faith, integrity, ambition).
2. **Visualize Your Ideal Relationship:** Find quotes, affirmations, or images that represent the kind of love and partnership you desire. Create a small vision board or save them in a digital file for inspiration.
3. **Write a Prayer or Affirmation for Your Future Partner:** Include gratitude for their qualities and how they will complement your growth and purpose. Read it regularly to keep your intentions clear and grounded.
4. **Evaluate Yourself:** Journal about how you can embody the qualities you're looking for in a partner. Focus on becoming the best version of yourself to attract the right relationship.

Reflections

_____

_____

_____

_____

_____

_____

_____

_____

_____

_____

_____

_____

_____

Reflections

_____

_____

_____

_____

_____

_____

_____

_____

_____

_____

_____

_____

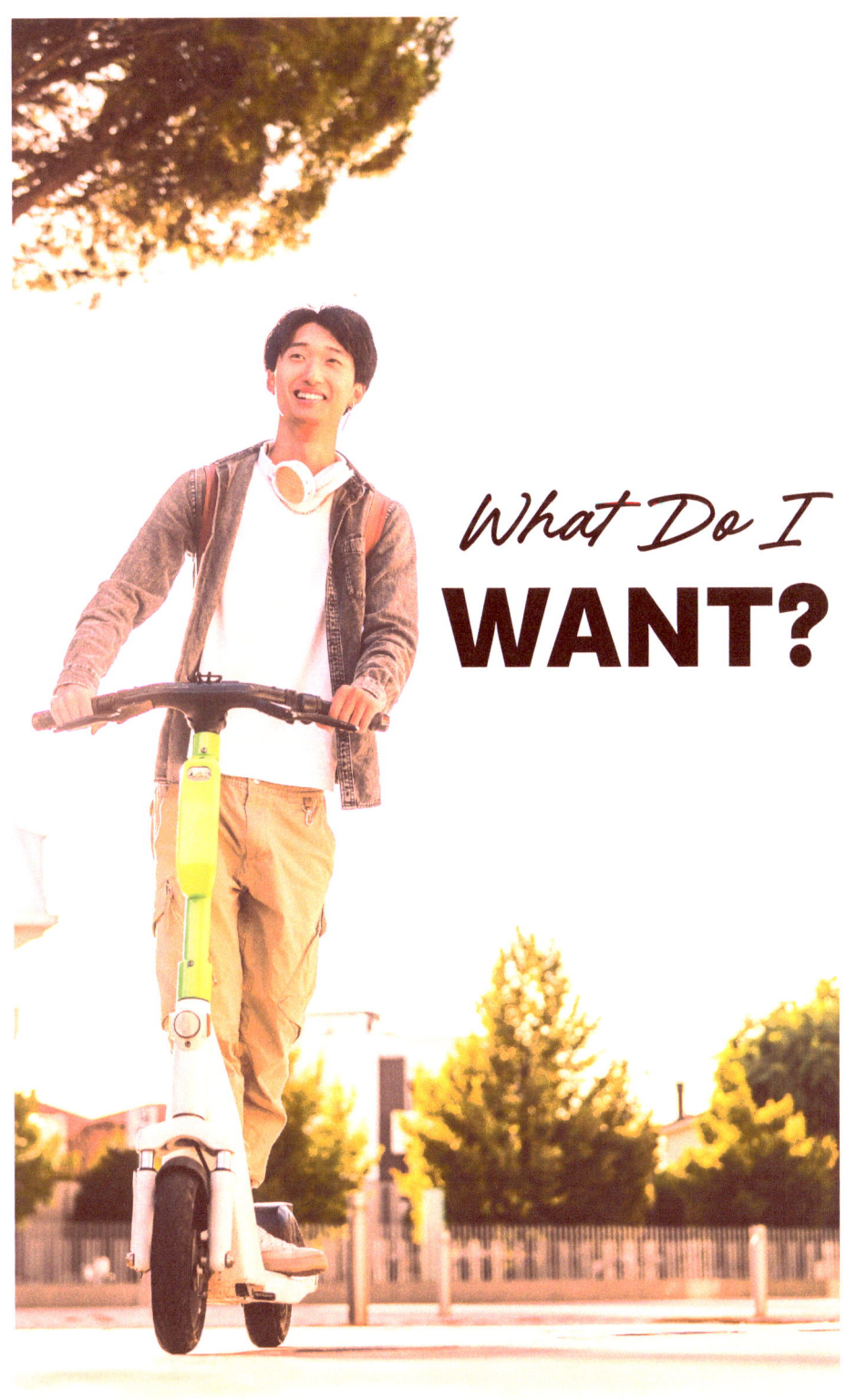

What Do I
WANT?

What Do I Want?

This is your time, a season to claim all you want, to tell God your new hearts desires. You would be silly to think for even a second that you won't get it. 2024 was an amazing year for me, so many business accomplishments, personally victories, but moreover healing with the help of God and very specific prayers.

And so here in 2025 I set out to be intentional, I wrote a list of all I am asking God to do and I am leaving it in His hands to open the doors while I take the action. So, dear friend, what do you want? Like really want, unapologetically, and know that it is yours for the claiming.

Questions for Reflection:

1. **Personal Values and Purpose:**
   - What values are most important to me right now?
   - What gives my life meaning and purpose?
2. **Relationships and Connection:**
   - What kind of relationships do I want in my life (romantic, friendships, family)?
   - How do I want to feel in my relationships?
3. **Career and Goals:**
   - What kind of work or projects excite me?
   - Where do I see myself in 1 year? 5 years?
4. **Lifestyle and Experiences:**
   - What does my ideal day look like?
   - What hobbies, activities, or adventures do I want to explore?
5. **Emotional and Spiritual Growth:**
   - How do I want to feel emotionally on a daily basis?
   - What role does faith, spirituality, or mindfulness play in my life?

6. **Legacy and Impact:**
   - What kind of impact do I want to leave on others?
   - How do I want to be remembered?

1. **Create a Vision Statement:**
   - Write a 1–2 paragraph statement describing the life you want to create—emotionally, spiritually, physically, and professionally.
2. **Make a 'Desires List':**
   - List 10 things you truly want, no matter how big or small, and prioritize them.
3. **Break It Down:**
   - Take your top 3 desires and create 1 small actionable step for each one to start working toward it this week.
4. **Visualize Your Future:**
   - Create a vision board (physical or digital) with images and words that represent what you want. Display it somewhere you'll see it daily.
5. **Daily Journaling Prompt:**
   - Each morning or evening, write one sentence starting with: "Today, I want to feel…" and track whether your actions align with that intention.
6. **Accountability Check-In:**
   - Set a date (weekly or monthly) to revisit your goals, track your progress, and adjust as needed.

Reflections

_____

_____

_____

_____

_____

_____

_____

_____

_____

_____

_____

_____

Reflections

_____

_____

_____

_____

_____

_____

_____

_____

_____

_____

_____

_____

Reflections

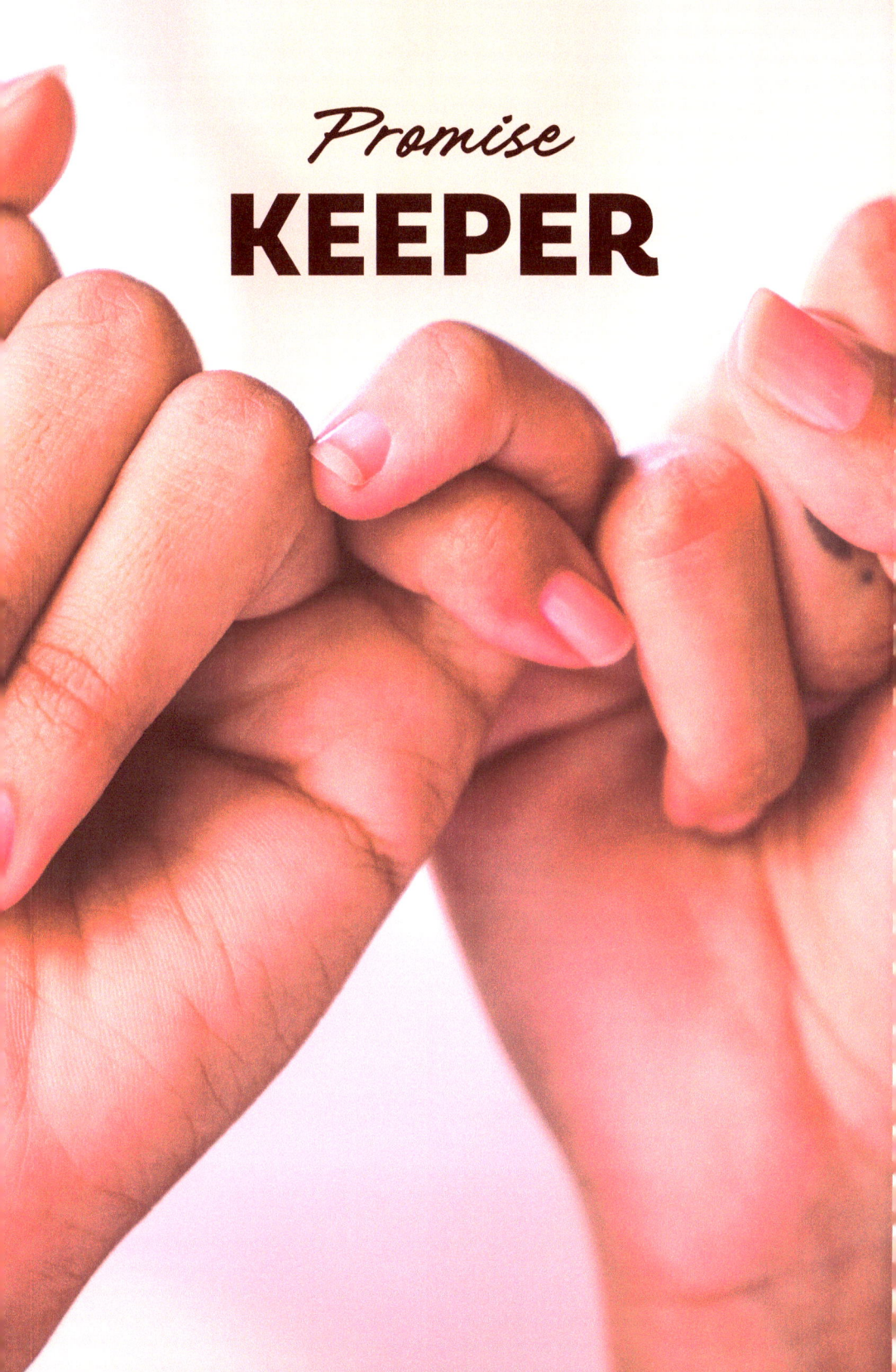

Promise Keeper

Now this one, is all on you. What promises are you going to keep to yourself going forward to maintain all the hard work you have done? Write a letter to yourself regarding what you will never allow again, and how you will show up for yourself this year.

This is a vow that no matter what, you will not repeat the same behaviors that did not honor the incredible person that you are in this world.

How can you approach future self-promises with greater intention and success?

_____

_____

_____

_____

_____

_____

_____

_____

Reflections

_____

_____

_____

_____

_____

_____

_____

_____

_____

_____

_____

Reflections

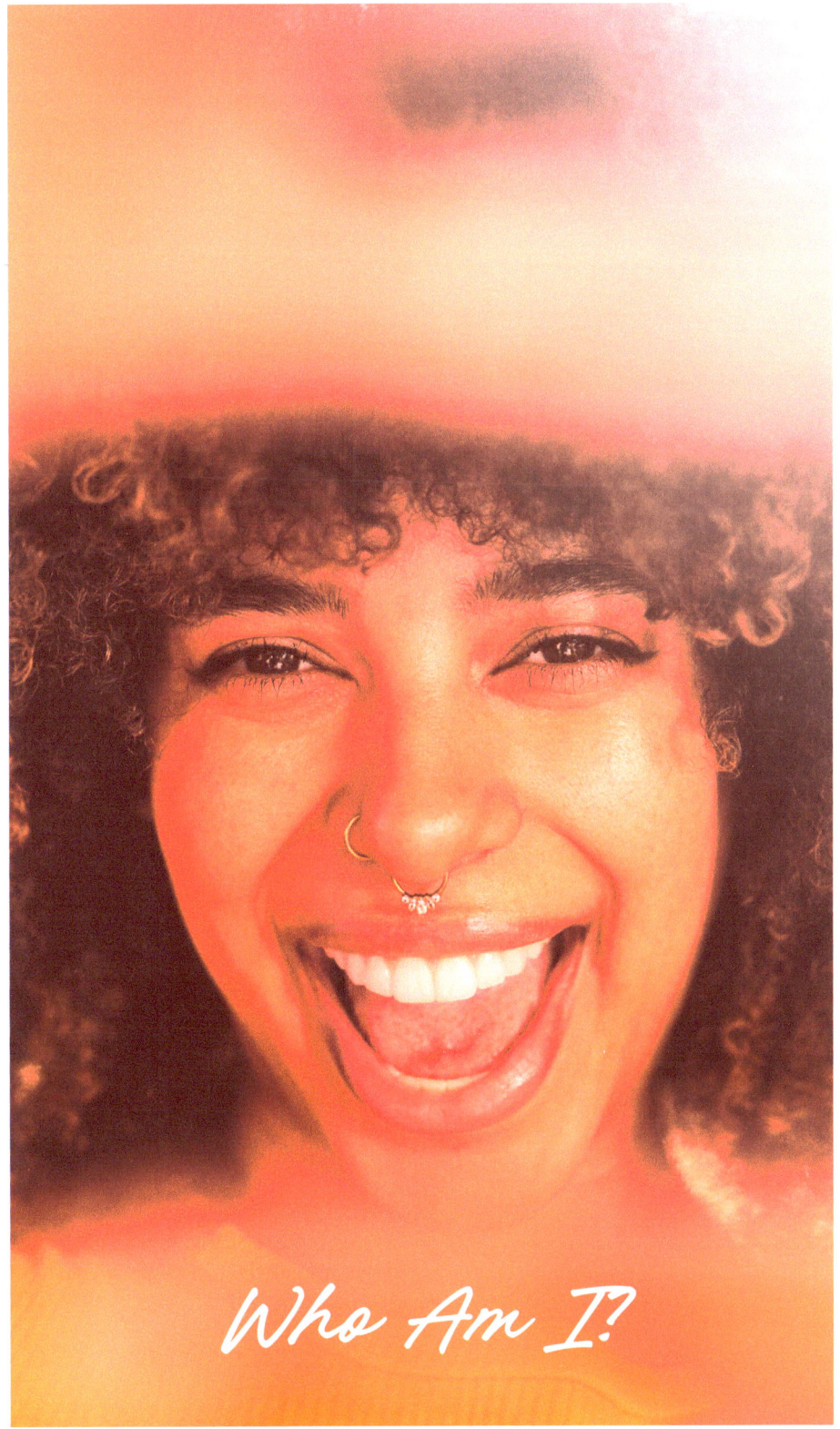

Who Am I?

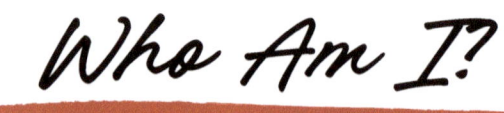

Who Am I?

I have found that in this world, so many outsiders, societal pressures attempt to label and tell us who we are, and who we aren't good enough to be. I chuckle at that notion, because sometimes we buy into it when really no one knows us like God, ourselves, and the people who truly care about us.

You are doing the work; you stuck through this workbook and have begun your healing. The journey is a forever one, and will have many turns and deep dives that continue to show you who you are. I believe it is imperative to know who God says we are, and how He sees us, as we are perfect in His sight. So, shedding the characteristics others bestowed upon you in a negative light, utilize the scriptures on page 90 to intentionally remind yourself of who you truly are.

Pick 5 or 6 and continue to add throughout your life's journey.

Thank you for allowing me to share space with you, remember that you have come so far from where you started. Be blessed.

Using the following pages, write 5-6 scriptures, starting from page 88 that highlight who you are.

Who Am I?

_____

_____

_____

_____

_____

_____

_____

_____

_____

_____

_____

_____

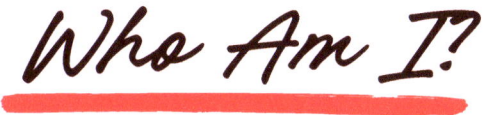

Who Am I?

I am faithful
(Ephesians 1:1)

I am blessed in the heavenly realms with every spiritual blessing
(Ephesians 1:3)

I am chosen before the creation of the world
(Ephesians 1:4, 11)

I am holy and blameless
(Ephesians 1:4)

I am adopted as his child
(Ephesians 1:5)

I am given Gods glorious grace lavishly and without restriction
(Ephesians 1:3)

I am in Him
(Ephesians 1:7)

I have redemption
(Ephesians 1:8)

I am forgiven
(Ephesians 1:8)

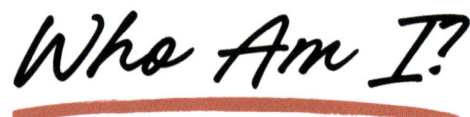

Who Am I?

I have purpose
(Ephesians 1:9 & 3:11)

I have hope
(Ephesians 1:12)

I am included
(Ephesians 1:13)

I am sealed with the promised Holy Spirit
(Ephesians 1:13)

I am a saint
(Ephesians 1:18)

I am alive with Christ
(Ephesians 2:5)

I am raised up with Christ
(Ephesians 2:6)

I am seated with Christ in the heavenly realms
(Ephesians 2:6)

I have been shown the incomparable riches of God's grace
(Ephesians 2:7)

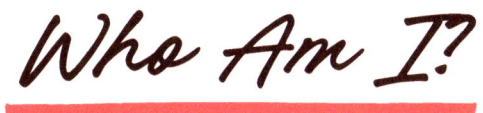
Who Am I?

God has expressed His kindness to me
(Ephesians 2:7)

I am God's workmanship
(Ephesians 2:10)

I have been brought near to God through Christ's blood **(Ephesians 2:13)**

I have peace
(Ephesians 2:14)

I have access to the Father
(Ephesians 2:18)

I am a member of God's household
(Ephesians 2:19)

I am secure
(Ephesians 2:20)

I am a holy temple
(Ephesians 2:21)

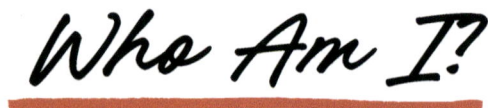
Who Am I?

I am a dwelling for the Holy Spirit
(Ephesians 2:22)

I share in the promise of Christ Jesus
(Ephesians 3:6)

God's power works through me
(Ephesians 3:7)

I can approach God with freedom and confidence
(Ephesians 3:12)

I know there is a purpose for my sufferings
(Ephesians 3:13)

I am completed by God
(Ephesians 3:19)

I have been called
(Ephesians 4: 1;2)

I can be humble, gentle, patient, and lovingly tolerant of others
(Ephesians 4:2)

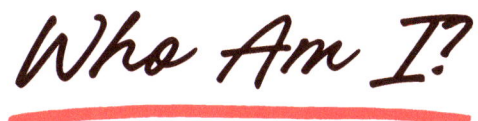
Who Am I?

I can mature spiritually
(Ephesians 4:15)

I can be certain of God's truths and the lifestyle
that He has called me to
(Ephesians 4:2)

I can have a new attitude and new lifestyle
(Ephesians 4:21-32)

I can be kind and compassionate to others
(Ephesians 4:32)

I can forgive others
(Ephesians 4:32)

I can give thanks for everything
(Ephesians 5:20)

I can be strong
(Ephesians 6:10)

I have God's power
(Ephesians 6:10)

www.ingramcontent.com/pod-product-compliance
Lightning Source LLC
Chambersburg PA
CBHW040856120626
46551CB00001B/49